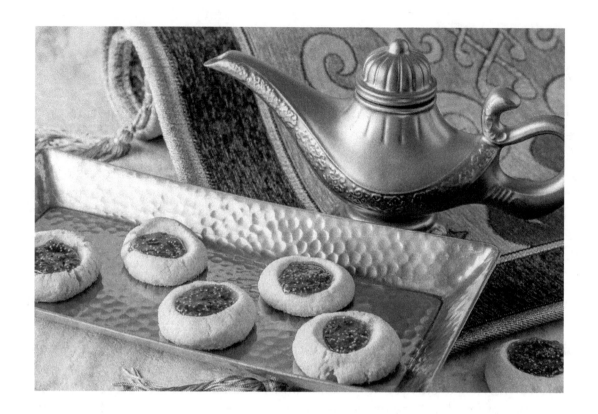

CONTENTS

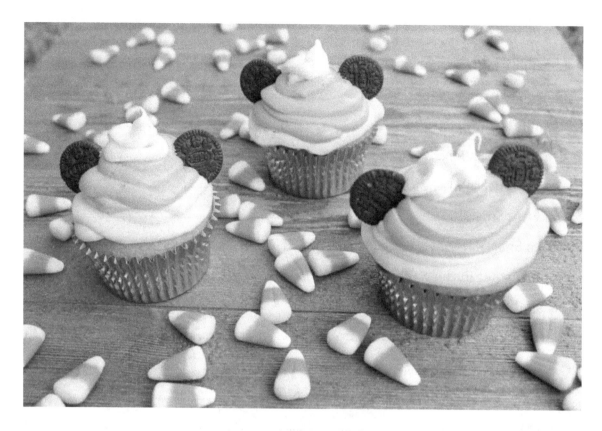

INTRODUCTION

Before you start cooking your first recipes, it is very important to learn a little bit about safety in the kitchen. While the kitchen is certainly a fun place, it is also full of dangerous tools that need to be handled with care. Here are a few safety tips for cooking in the kitchen with kids.

1. Use the Oven with Care

Ovens help cook our foods and are a very important kitchen tool. However, ovens are extremely hot and can easily burn you if you are not careful. Younger kids should never be allowed to use the oven and should learn early on that they are not to touch the oven or the oven door. When cooking with younger kids, adults should be in charge of putting foods in and out of the oven. When an adult opens the oven door, the kids should all stand a few feet away. This will prevent the kids from getting to close by accident or having the hot air hit them when the oven is first opened. If kids are very anxious to see how their food is cooking, utilize the oven light. Most ovens have an interior light and a glass door so your can peer in and see the food as it bakes. Kids will definitely find it fun to see inside the oven and watch the food cook and it is much safer than allowing them to touch the oven.

Once old enough, kids should still use the oven with care (and adults too!). When opening the hot oven door, always have a pot holder handy just in case you need to reach in and pull something out. Buy pot holders that are specifically for oven use (not decorative) and can withstand high temperatures. When kids first start using the oven, you may want to purchase a set of oven mitts that they can put their entire hand and forearm into, protecting their hands and arms fully as they reach in the hot oven.

When using the oven to cook, always preheat it to the temperature needed, turning it on about 15 minutes before you begin cooking. This will ensure that the oven is at the correct temperature to cook the food. Also, be sure to turn the oven off when you are done!

2. Stovetop Burners

Cooking food on the stove can also be dangerous for kids. When cooking with younger kids, adults should do all the stovetop cooking, letting the kids measure and stir when the stove is hot. For older kids, make sure they learn about stovetop safety.

One thing to remember is that not only is the burner very hot, but the pan holding the food is also quite hot. Touching either can result in injury. If you are stirring with a metal spoon while cooking over a burner, the spoon can also get hot. A good tip is to wear flexible oven mitts while cooking over the stove to keep your hands and arms protected. You should also always choose heat resistant utensils and pans that have heat resistant handles, allowing you to touch them without getting burned.

If possible, invest in a small induction burner for kids to use when learning how to cook. Induction burners heat pans with magnets which spin under a glass surface. There is no open flame and no hot coils. The surface of the burner does get hot but not nearly as hot as a traditional gas or electric stovetop. You can purchase a single induction burner that can be kept in a cabinet and pulled out whenever your kids are ready to cook!

3. Knifes

Many recipes require chopping or cutting food. Once again, adults should do these steps for younger kids, slicing, chopping and cutting anything needed for the recipe. Once the kids start being of an age where they are able to handle a knife, look for a kids safety knife and cutting board set. These knifes are not nearly as sharp as regular knifes and are a perfect way for kids to learn safe knife skills.

When kids begin using knives, teach them to always keep the blade of the knife facing down toward the cutting board. When they pick up the knife, only touch the handle and, again, keep the blade facing downward. Slice slowly and carefully- cooking is never a race and there is safety in taking your time! If you are holding a food while you cut it, move your hand when the knife starts to get

close to your fingers. It is okay to discard a small piece of food that was too tricky to cut safely. If you ever drop a knife in the kitchen, let it fall to the floor- do not try to catch it! You do not want to catch a knife the wrong way and end up injured. It is much easier to let the knife fall, wash it and keep on cooking!

4. Wash Your Hands

One of the most important tips in food safety is proper hand washing. Before you start cooking, everyone who will be involved in the cooking process should wash their hands with warm, soapy water. This will help prevent the spread of germs and keep the food you are about to make safe!

As you cook, wash your hands immediately anytime you touch raw meat in order to prevent cross contamination (that means when germs from one food gets on to another food- meats and seafood have the most germs so you should be extra careful when handling these!). You should also just wash your hands anytime they get messy. The more you wash your hands, the better!

5. Ask Permission

Kids can be anxious to start cooking right away, anytime that dream of being a chef hits them! However, kids should always ask permission before they start cooking so that adults are aware of what they are doing in the kitchen. Sometimes, a kid may want to make a recipe that is a little more advanced and they will help so they should ask! One good idea is to place this recipe book up high, on a shelf where your kids can't quite reach it. When they are ready to cook, they will need to ask you to get the book, also informing you that cooking is about to commence!

Kids should also always ask permission before taste testing a recipe. Food is delicious, we all want to eat it! But it also needs to be safe to eat. There are plenty of recipes where it is perfectly okay to try the food you are cooking as you move through the recipe. However, there are other recipes that are not okay to try until they are completely done. Testing anything with raw meat, for example, is not a good idea. Kids may not know what is safe to try and what is not so train them to ask before they lick! In addition, always do a taste test with a clean spoon or utensil and then set it aside to be cleaned. This will prevent spreading germs!

6. Food Safety

In addition to keeping our bodies safe when in the kitchen, it is also important to keep the food we are making safe. Some foods are not safe to eat before they are cooked. One perfect example is raw meat which needs to be cooked to a certain temperature to kill harmful bacteria inside the meat. Younger kids should never be allowed to handle raw meat and older kids should learn about proper food handling. This includes cutting raw meats on their own cutting board then washing it with soap and hot water afterward. After handling raw meat, hands should always be washed along with any utensils and countertops that the raw meat may have touched. Taking the time to handle foods properly is essential to making food that is safe to eat.

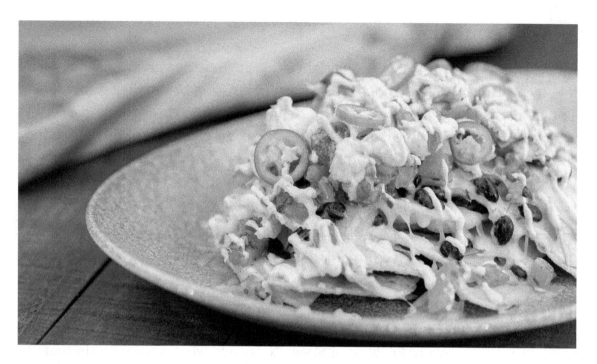

THINGS KIDS CAN DO IN THE KITCHEN

There are plenty of things that kids can help with in the kitchen, even when they are just old enough to hold a spoon! While there are no set ages when kids are able to complete certain cooking tasks, parents should use their best judgement when deciding if a certain task is something their kids can handle. There are several recipes inside this book that require using the oven, cutting vegetables or cooking on the stovetop. An adult should look over the recipe and decide which tasks the kids will be able to do and which they will need help with. However, there are always ways to involve kids, no matter how challenging the recipe! Take a look at the following things all kids can do in the kitchen.

1. Measuring

Kids are great at measuring ingredients which is perfect as every, single recipe needs to be measured! With younger kids, an adult can hand them the correct measurement and simply have them scoop the ingredient into the bowl. Older kids will be able to measure on their own, also learning about different volumes of foods and fractions.

2. Mixing

Kids of all ages are good at mixing. For younger kids, give them a large bowl than needed so that when they wildly mix, all the ingredients stay inside the bowl. An adult may need to give the ingredients and extra mix or two after the younger kids have had their turn to really blend the ingredients well! Older kids should be able to mix everything on their own and learn about different mixing tools as they go. A whisk, a wooden spoon and a rubber spatula all mix foods differently!

3. Tasting

While tasting foods as you cook is mentioned in our kitchen safety guidelines above, it is also one of the most fun parts of cooking. Let the kids taste the foods as they cook (as long as it is safe and they have asked permission!), trying the

food at every stage of the recipe. They will learn how various ingredients interact to change the taste of a food. They will also expand their pallet, trying new things an discovering new food loves.

4. Gather Ingredients

A great kitchen task for kids is to collect all the ingredients needed for a recipe. When the kids are still too young to read, an adult can ask for each ingredient and help the kids find it in the kitchen. Older kids should be able to do this on their own. Older kids can also help write grocery lists, looking at a recipe, assessing what they need versus what they have and writing down a list of necessities. Ingredient identification and kitchen organization is key to cooking and this can be taught from a very young age!

5. Preparing pans

Many recipes ask for a greased sheet tray, a greased muffin tin or a paper lined sheet tray. Let the kids spray the grease, spread the butter on the pan and rip the parchment paper to line the tray. These are all great activities for kids of all ages.

6. Skewer Foods

Kids love foods on a stick so why not also let them put the food on the stick. Making kebobs and pushing popsicle sticks into foods are both easy things kids can do in the kitchen. There is no sharp tools or hot appliances involved!

7. Cleaning Up

No matter the age, kids can be involved in cleaning up the kitchen after making a recipe. Putting away ingredients, putting bowls in the sink and wiping counters are all suitable for kids of any age. Once kids are a little older, they should be able to wash, dry and put away all the tools they used to make a recipe. A clean kitchen is essential to making good foods!

As you can see, cooking is a skill that everyone can learn, no matter what their age. So whether you are a mom to a two year old who wants to have her child help in the kitchen or a teen who is ready to start whipping up their own recipes, this book is for you! Pick any recipe in here and you are guaranteed to create a delicious, fun, healthy meal!

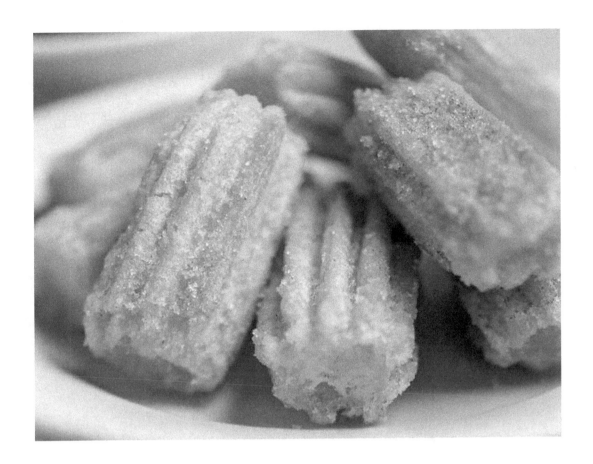

Breakfast

Banana Pancakes

Preparation Time: 5 minutes

Cooking Time: 5 minutes

Servings: 4 servings

Ingredients

- 2 ripe bananas
- 4 eggs
- 1 tsp vanilla extract
- ¼ tsp baking powder
- 1 pinch salt
- 4 tsp coconut oil or butter

Instructions

1. Place the bananas in a large bowl and sprinkle the baking powder and salt over them.
2. Use a fork to mash the bananas well. They should be as smooth as possible. However, a few banana pieces are okay.
3. Add the vanilla extract and eggs to the bowl and stir everything together well. The eggs should be fully incorporated into the batter.
4. Pour 1 teaspoon of the coconut oil into a small sauce pan and heat over medium heat.
5. Add ¼ of the batter to the pan and let cook for 2-3 minutes.
6. Flip the pancake and cook for one more minute.
7. Remove the pancake from the pan and serve with your kids favorite toppings (syrup, fresh fruit or whipped cream).
8. Repeat the cooking process with the remaining pancake batter.

Nutrition: Calories 171, fat 9g, fiber 2g, carbs 15g, protein 7g

Yogurt Parfait

Preparation Time: 5 minutes

Cooking Time: 0 minutes

Servings: 2 servings

Ingredients:

- 2 cups vanilla yogurt
- 1 cup strawberries, chopped
- ½ cup blueberries
- ½ cup raspberries
- 2 Tbsp honey

Instructions

1. Divide the chopped strawberries between two clear glasses. For older kids, use glass but for younger kids, choose a plastic cup that is clear or opaque.
2. Top the strawberries with 1/3 cup of yogurt in each glass.
3. Divide the blueberries between each glass then top each with another 1/3 cup yogurt.
4. Add the raspberries to each glass and then top with the remaining yogurt.
5. Drizzle one tablespoon of honey over each glass and serve!

Nutrition: Calories 221, fat 2g, fiber 7g, carbs 58g, protein 8g

Donut Apples

Preparation Time: 10 minutes

Cooking Time: 0 minutes

Servings: 2 servings

Ingredients:

- 2 Apples, cores removed
- ½ cup cream cheese
- Rainbow Sprinkles

Instructions

1. Slice the donuts horizontally so each slice has a hole in the center where the core was removed. The slices should look like donuts!
2. Spread a thin layer of cream cheese across each apple slice.
3. Sprinkle each slice with the rainbow sprinkles and serve! These donut apples are best when served right away.

*Note:

You can dye the cream cheese frosting with food coloring to make pretty donut "icing". You can also blend fresh strawberries, fresh blueberries or blackberries into the cream cheese to flavor it.

Nutrition: Calories 403, fat 26g, fiber 5g, carbs 43g, protein 4g

Cinnamon French Toast

Preparation Time: 5 minutes

Cooking Time: 6 minutes

Servings: 4 servings

Ingredients:

- 4 slices whole wheat bread
- 1 egg
- ½ cup whole milk
- 1 tsp cinnamon
- 2 tbsp maple syrup
- 1 tsp vanilla extract
- 4 tsp coconut oil or butter

Instructions

1. In a large bowl, whisk the egg, milk, cinnamon, syrup and vanilla together well.
2. Add 1 tsp of coconut oil to a small saute pan and heat over medium.
3. Dip one piece of bread into the egg mixture, covering it completely and then place it right into the hot pan.
4. Cook for 2 minutes and then flip the bread over, cooking for 2 more minutes.
5. Remove the French toast from the pan and repeat, cooking the remaining French toast with the same method. Serve hot with your favorite toppings (strawberries, whipped cream, ice cream, or syrup).

Nutrition: Calories 174, fat 9g, fiber 2g, carbs 28g, protein 7g

French Toast Muffins

Preparation Time: 10 minutes

Cooking Time: 30 minutes

Servings: 5 servings

Ingredients

- 4 slices whole wheat bread
- 3 eggs
- ¾ cup whole milk
- ¼ cup maple syrup
- 1 tsp cinnamon
- 1 tsp vanilla extract

Instructions

1. Preheat your oven to 350 degrees F.
2. In a large bowl, whisk the eggs, milk, syrup, cinnamon and vanilla. Beat until well combined.
3. Slice the bread into small 1 inch pieces and add to the egg mixture. Mix together well and set aside to allow the bread to soak for 5 minutes.
4. Spray a muffin tin with baking grease and then scoop the French toast mixture into each muffin cup, filling them about ¾ of the way full.
5. Place the muffin tin in the oven and bake for 30 minutes or until the muffins spring back to the touch.
6. Remove from the oven and let cool for 10 minutes. Serve warm

Nutrition: Calories 314, fat 5g, fiber 2g, carbs 58g, protein 8g

Waffle Popsicles

Preparation Time: 5 minutes

Cooking Time: 10 minutes

Servings: 4 servings

Ingredients:

- 1 egg
- 1 cup flour
- 1 cup whole milk
- ¼ cup vegetable oil
- 1 tsp vanilla extract
- 2 tsp sugar
- 2 tsp baking powder
- 1 pinch salt
- ¼ cup peanut butter
- ¼ cup chocolate chips

Instructions:

1. In a large bowl, whisk the egg, milk, oil, and vanilla extract together.
2. Add the flour, baking powder, sugar and salt. Whisk until a smooth batter forms.
3. Pour the batter into your preheated waffle iron, adding as much as your manufacturers directions instruct (typically about ½ cup batter in a standard waffle iron).
4. Cook until golden brown, again based on your manufacturers directions.
5. Remove the waffle from the pan and let cool. Cook the remaining batter.
6. Cut each waffle into four equal pieces and stick a popsicle stick into each piece.
7. Drizzle each waffle pop with the peanut butter and sprinkle with chocolate chips. Serve!

*Note: Drizzle the waffle pops with melted chocolate and top with sprinkles for an extra special treat.

Nutrition: Calories 459, fat 27g, fiber 3g, carbs 44g, protein 11g

PBJ Waffles

Preparation Time: 10 minutes

Cooking Time: 10 minutes

Servings: 4 servings

Ingredients:

- 1 egg
- 1 cup flour
- 1 cup whole milk
- ¼ cup vegetable oil
- 1 tsp vanilla extract
- 2 tsp sugar
- 2 tsp baking powder
- 1 pinch salt
- ½ cup peanut butter
- ½ cup strawberry Jelly

Instructions:

1. In a large bowl, whisk the egg, milk, oil, and vanilla extract together.
2. Add the flour, baking powder, sugar and salt. Whisk until a smooth batter forms.
3. Pour the batter into your preheated waffle iron, adding as much as your manufacturers directions instruct (typically about ½ cup batter in a standard waffle iron).
4. Cook until golden brown, again based on your manufacturers directions.
5. Remove the waffle from the pan and let cool. Cook the remaining batter- you should get 4 large waffles.
6. Spread the peanut butter on two of the waffles and the jelly on the other two waffles. Sandwich one peanut butter and one jelly waffle together then cut into pieces. Serve for breakfast!

Nutrition: Calories 504, fat 34g, fiber 3g, carbs 67g, protein 14g

Yogurt Popsicles

Preparation Time: 5 minutes

Cooking Time: 0 minutes

Servings: 4 servings

Ingredients:

- 2 cups vanilla yogurt
- ½ cup slices strawberries
- 1 kiwi, sliced
- ¼ cup blueberries, sliced

Instructions:

1. Have a large popsicle mold on hand with at least 4 popsicle cavities.
2. Add a little yogurt to the bottom of each popsicle mold.
3. Add about half of the fruit slices to the molds, dividing evenly.
4. Add a little more yogurt to cover the fruit.
5. Add remaining fruit into the molds and finish with the rest of the yogurt.
6. Place a popsicle stick into each pop and freeze until set (about 4 hours).
7. Serve frozen as a great breakfast treat!

Nutrition: Calories 147, fat 1g, fiber 3g, carbs 34g, protein 4g

Banana Pops

Preparation Time: 10 minutes

Cooking Time: 0 minutes

Servings: 4 servings

Ingredients:

- 4 ripe bananas
- ½ cup granola
- ¼ cup chocolate chips

Instructions:

1. Peel each banana and place a popsicle stick into the end of each, making 4 big pops.
2. Mix the granola and the chocolate chips together on a sheet tray, breaking up the granola into small pieces. You don't want any large clumps.
3. Roll each banana in the granola mix, covering the outside of the banana in the granola and chocolate chips. You may need to press down slightly to get the granola to stick but it should stay on pretty well on it's own.
4. Serve immediately!

*Notes:

-For smaller kids, cut the banana in half to make it more manageable on a stick

Nutrition: Calories 245, fat 6g, fiber 5g, carbs 47g, protein 4g

Egg Flowers

Preparation Time: 10 minutes

Cooking Time: 8 minutes

Servings: 4 servings

Ingredients:

- 1 Bell Pepper
- 1 tomato
- 4 eggs
- ¼ tsp salt
- 1/8 tsp ground black pepper
- 2 Tbsp olive oil

Instructions:

1. Remove the stem and seeds from the center of a bell pepper, using a sharp knife to cut around the stem and pop out the center.
2. Slice the bell pepper horizontally so you get 4 circular, hollow slices.
3. Slice the tomato into four slices as well.
4. Add the oil to a saute pan and heat over medium.
5. Place the pepper slices into the pan and place a tomato slice inside each pepper slice, making a little "cup".
6. Crack one egg into each pepper cup, keeping the yolk whole.
7. Cover the pan and cook the egg flowers for about 8 minutes or until the egg is set to your liking.
8. Use a spatula to remove each flower from the pan and place on a plate.
9. Sprinkle with salt and pepper. Enjoy while hot!

Nutrition: Calories 150, fat 12g, fiber 1g, carbs 5g, protein 7g

Mini Breakfast Burritos

Preparation Time: 10 minutes

Cooking Time: 5 minutes

Servings: 2 servings

Ingredients:

- 2 Eggs
- ¼ cup whole milk
- 2 whole wheat tortillas
- ¼ cup grated cheese
- ¼ tsp salt
- 1/8 tsp ground black pepper
- 2 tbsp butter or olive oil

Instructions:

1. In a small bowl, whisk together the eggs, milk, salt, pepper and cheese.
2. Add 1 tbsp of the butter into a small saute pan and heat over medium.
3. Add half the egg mixture to the pan and cover. Cook for 4 minutes or until the eggs are set.
4. Use a spatula to remove the eggs from the pan and slide on top of one of the tortillas.
5. While hot, roll the tortilla tightly and set aside.
6. Cook the remaining egg, repeating the cooking process.
7. Slice both tortilla roll ups into small, bite sized circles. Serve warm

Nutrition: Calories 448, fat 37g, fiber 4g, carbs 38g, protein 24g

Open Faced Banana Sandwich

Preparation Time: 8 minutes

Cooking Time: 0 minutes

Servings: 2 servings

Ingredients:

- 2 ripe bananas
- ½ cup almond butter
- ¼ cup raisins
- 4 Tbsp honey
- ¼ cup crushed almonds
- ¼ cup mini chocolate chips

Instructions:

1. Slice each banana in half lengthwise and place two slices on each plate.
2. Divide the almond butter between each banana slice, carefully spreading it across the length of the banana.
3. Drizzle one tablespoon of honey over each banana slice, on top of the almond butter.
4. Sprinkle each banana with raisins, almonds and chocolate chips.
5. Enjoy chilled or room temperature, with a fork or by hand!

Nutrition: Calories 503, fat 24g, fiber 13g, carbs 124g, protein 15g

Apple Pie Oatmeal

Preparation Time: 5 minutes

Cooking Time: 5 minutes

Servings: 2 servings

Ingredients:

- 1 apple, diced
- 2 Tbsp water
- 1 Tbsp honey
- ½ tsp vanilla extract
- 1 tsp cinnamon
- ¼ tsp nutmeg
- ½ tsp cornstarch
- 1 cup oatmeal, cooked

Instructions:

1. Combine the apples, water, honey, and vanilla together in a small pot. Stir together briefly.
2. Sprinkle the apples with he cornstarch and then bring to a boil over medium heat, stirring occasionally.
3. Boil for about 2 minutes or until thickened.
4. Stir in the cinnamon and nutmeg.
5. Serve apple pie filling over the cooked oatmeal and enjoy warm.

Nutrition: Calories 128, fat 1g, fiber 4g, carbs 29g, protein 1g

Egg Mufins

Preparation Time: 20 minutes

Cooking Time: 30 minutes

Servings: 4 servings

Ingredients:

- 2 eggs
- ¼ cup whole milk
- ½ cup shredded cheese
- ¼ cup chopped tomatoes
- ¼ cup bacon, chopped
- ¼ tsp salt
- 1/8 tsp ground black pepper
- ¼ tsp paprika

Instructions:

1. In a small bowl, whisk together the eggs and milk.
2. Add the cheese, salt, pepper and paprika and whisk.
3. Add the tomatoes and bacon and stir.
4. Spray a mini muffin pan with baking grease and preheat your oven to 375 degrees F.
5. Scoop the egg mix into the muffin cups, making sure each cup gets some egg and bacon. Fill the cups about ¾ of the way full.
6. Bake the mini muffins for about 30 minutes or until the tops begin to brown slightly.
7. Remove from the oven and serve warm.

Nutrition: Calories 166, fat 12g, fiber 1g, carbs 4g, protein 11g

Chocolate Zucchini Bread

Preparation Time: 10 minutes

Cooking Time: 10 minutes

Servings: 5 servings

Ingredients:

- 1 egg
- 2 Tbsp applesauce
- 2 Tbsp honey
- 1 tsp vanilla extract
- ¼ cup brown sugar
- ½ tsp baking soda
- ¾ tsp baking powder
- ¼ cup cocoa powder
- ½ cup grated zucchini
- ¾ cup flour
- 1/3 cup mini chocolate chips

Instructions:

1. In a large bowl, combine the egg, applesauce, honey and vanilla extract and stir.
2. Stir in the zucchini.
3. Add the remaining ingredients and mix well.
4. Pour the batter into a greased loaf pan then place into a preheated 374 degree F oven.
5. Bake for 40 minutes and check. If a toothpick come out of the center cleanly, the bread is done.
6. Remove from the oven, allow to cool and then remove the loaf from the pan.
7. Slice and serve!

Nutrition: Calories 350, fat 4g, fiber 7g, carbs 41g, protein 8g

Egg Recipes

Simple Cheesy Eggs

Preparation Time: 5 minutes

Cooking Time: 5 minutes

Servings: 2 servings

Ingredients:

- 4 eggs
- 2 Tbsp whole milk
- ¼ tsp salt
- Ground black pepper
- ½ cup shredded cheddar cheese
- 1 Tbsp butter

Instructions:

1. In a small bowl, whisk together the eggs, milk, salt and pepper. Whisk until well blended.
2. Stir the cheddar cheese into the mix.
3. Add the butter to a small sauce pan and heat over medium.
4. Once the butter has melted, pour the egg mixture into the pan and cook for 4 minutes, stirring constantly.
5. Move the hot eggs to a plate and serve.

Nutrition: Calories 343, fat 27g, fiber 0g, carbs 4g, protein 21g

Egg Pops

Preparation Time: 10 minutes

Cooking Time: 10 minutes

Servings: 4 servings

Ingredients:

- 1 carrot, peeled
- 1 celery stalk
- 8 eggs, hard boiled

Instructions:

1. Cut the carrot into 4 large carrot sticks. Trim them so that they are about 4 inches long.
2. Cut the celery stalk into 4 pieces as well, each stick being about 4 inches long.
3. Stick one celery stick or one carrot stick into all of the eggs, making an egg pop!
4. Serve with a sprinkle of salt and pepper or serve with dip like hummus or guacamole.

Nutrition: Calories 149, fat 10g, fiber 0g, carbs 2g, protein 13g

Breakfast Pizza

Preparation Time: 5 minutes

Cooking Time: 15 minutes

Servings: 2 servings

Ingredients:

- 4 eggs, whisked
- 1 Tbsp butter or olive oil
- 1/2 cup pizza sauce
- 2 plain or whole wheat English muffins
- ½ cup shredded mozzarella cheese

Instructions:

1. Add the butter to a small skillet and heat over medium. Add the whisked eggs and let cook, unstirred for 2 minutes. Break the eggs up slightly with a spatula, leaving large pieces. Turn off heat.
2. Break each English muffin in half and spread 2 Tbsp of pizza sauce across the top of each slice.
3. Place the eggs on top of the pizza sauce, dividing the eggs evenly between each English muffin.
4. Sprinkle with the mozzarella cheese.
5. Place the English muffins on a lined sheet tray and put them into a preheated 450 degree oven. Cook for 5 minutes.
6. Remove from the oven and serve warm.

Nutrition: Calories 198, fat 9g, fiber 1g, carbs 16g, protein 13g

Coffee Cup Scrambled Eggs

Preparation Time: 1 minutes

Cooking Time: 2 minutes

Servings: 1 servings

Ingredients:

- ½ cup shredded hash browns, frozen
- 1 large egg
- 1 Tbsp milk
- 2 Tbsp shredded cheese

Instructions:

1. Find a mug that is microwave safe and spray the inside of the mug with cooking spray.
2. Add the hash browns to the bottom of the cup.
3. Add the egg and milk on top of the hash browns and whisk together gently until nicely blended.
4. Microwave on high for 30 seconds then stir and microwave for another 30 seconds.
5. Sprinkle the cheese on top of the hot eggs and enjoy!

Nutrition: Calories 201, fat 3g, fiber 1g, carbs 16g, protein 11g

Easy Egg Tortilla

Preparation Time: 1 minutes

Cooking Time: 2 minutes

Servings: 1 servings

Ingredients:

- 1 large egg
- 1 piece of cooked breakfast sausage, chopped
- 2 Tbsp shredded cheddar cheese
- 1 whole wheat tortilla

Instructions:

1. Find a microwave safe cereal bowl or any bowl with a large, flatter bottom. Spray with cooking spray.
2. Add the egg to the bowl and whisk until it is well blended. Add the sausage and stir gently.
3. Microwave the egg and sausage mix for 45 seconds, stir then microwave again for another 20 seconds.
4. Use a spatula to move the eggs to the tortilla. Sprinkle with cheese and then fold in half or roll up. Enjoy while warm.

Nutrition: Calories 275, fat 6g, fiber 1g, carbs 18g, protein 13g

Microwave Flatbread Breakfast Pizza

Preparation Time: 1 minutes

Cooking Time: 2 minutes

Servings: 1 servings

Ingredients:

- 1 egg, whisked
- 2 Tbsp whole milk
- 2 Tbsp cooked breakfast sausage, chopped small
- 1 flatbread (or whole wheat tortilla)
- 2 Tbsp shredded mozzarella

Instructions:

1. Find a microwave safe cereal bowl or any bowl with a large, flatter bottom. Spray with cooking spray.
2. Add the egg to the bowl and whisk until it is well blended. Add the sausage and stir gently.
3. Microwave the egg and sausage mix for 45 seconds, stir then microwave again for another 20 seconds.
4. Move the eggs to the flatbread and sprinkle with the shredded cheese.
5. Cut into 4 "pizza" slices. Serve while warm

Nutrition: Calories 301, fat 5g, fiber 1g, carbs 20g, protein 17g

Eggs in a Nest

Preparation Time: 10 minutes

Cooking Time: 20 minutes

Servings: 4 servings

Ingredients:

- 2 cups shredded hash browns
- 1 cup shredded cheddar cheese
- 4 eggs
- ¼ tsp salt
- ¼ tsp ground black pepper

Instructions:

1. Mix the hash browns and cheese together in a small bowl.
2. Divide the hash brown and cheese mix between 4 greased ramekins. Press the mix up the sides of the ramekins slightly, making an indent in the center of the hash browns.
3. Place the ramekins into the oven for 10 minutes. Remove and crack one egg into each ramekin. Return the ramekins to the oven and bake for another 10 minutes.
4. Sprinkle with salt and pepper and serve while hot.

Nutrition: Calories 215, fat 12g, fiber 1g, carbs 7g, protein 13g

Egg and Cheese Waffles

Preparation Time: 5 minutes

Cooking Time: 15 minutes

Servings: 1 servings

Ingredients:

- 2 frozen waffles
- 1 egg, whisked
- ¼ cup shredded cheddar cheese

Instructions:

1. Place the waffles on a baking sheet and preheat your oven to 400 degrees F.
2. Slowly pour the whisked egg over the waffles, filling the waffle cavities with the whisked egg.
3. Place the tray in the oven and bake for 10 minutes.
4. Sprinkle one waffle with the cheddar cheese and then place the other waffle on top, making a sandwich. Let the sandwich sit for one minute to let the cheese melt and then enjoy.

Nutrition: Calories 299, fat 7g, fiber 1g, carbs 29g, protein 15g

Love Toast

Preparation Time: 5 minutes

Cooking Time: 15 minutes

Servings: 2 servings

Ingredients:

- 2 slices whole wheat bread
- 2 tsp butter
- 2 eggs
- ¼ tsp salt
- Pinch of pepper

Instructions:

1. Use a heart cutter to cut out a heart from the center of each piece of bread. Save the heart bread shapes.
2. Add the butter to a small skillet (that is large enough to fit two pieces of bread). Heat over medium heat to melt the butter.
3. Toast the bread and the heart cut outs in the skillet, making each side golden brown.
4. Crack one egg into the center heart of each piece of bread. Cover the pan and lower the heat to low.
5. Cook for about 10 minutes or until the egg whites are set.
6. Remove the bread and eggs from the pan and onto two plates. Sprinkle with the salt and pepper and serve with the heart cut outs.

Nutrition: Calories 180, fat 10g, fiber 1g, carbs 12g, protein 10g

Eggy Oatmeal

Preparation Time: 1 minute

Cooking Time: 3 minutes

Servings: 1 servings

Ingredients:

- 1 large egg
- 1/3 cup whole milk
- 1 package of instant oatmeal, maple or cinnamon raisin flavor
- ¼ cup Greek yogurt, plain or vanilla

Instructions:

1. In a microwave safe bowl, mix together the egg, milk and oatmeal packet.
2. Microwave the oatmeal mix on high for 2 minutes.
3. Remove from the microwave and top with the yogurt. Serve while warm

Nutrition: Calories 292, fat 3g, fiber 3g, carbs 36g, protein 13g

Vegetable Recipes

Green Bean Fries

Preparation Time: 5 minutes

Cooking Time: 15 minutes

Servings: 2 servings

Ingredients:

- ½ pound fresh green beans, ends sniped off
- 3 Tbsp chickpea hummus
- ½ cup bread crumbs
- ¼ cup shredded parmesan cheese

Instructions:

1. Place the hummus on a plate and the bread crumbs on a separate plate. Add the shredded cheese to the plate with the breadcrumbs and mix together gently.
2. Roll each green bean in the hummus and then in the breadcrumbs and place on a lined sheet tray.
3. Once all the beans are coated in the hummus and breadcrumbs, place in a preheated 400 degree oven for 15 minutes or until golden brown. Serve warm!

Nutrition: Calories 109, fat 8g, fiber 6g, carbs 30g, protein 12g

Rainbow Veggie Skewers

Preparation Time: 5 minutes

Cooking Time: 0 minutes

Servings: 2 servings

Ingredients:

- 4 cherry tomatoes
- 4 golden cherry tomatoes
- 4 pieces of broccoli
- 4 slices green bell pepper
- 4 baby purple carrots
- 4 pieces purple cauliflower

Instructions:

1. Grab 4 skewers, about 6 inches long.
2. Place one of each veggie on each skewer in the order listed to create a rainbow.
3. Serve chilled or room temperature, alone or with your favorite dip.

Nutrition: Calories 76, fat 0g, fiber 4g, carbs 18g, protein 2g

Spinach Balls

Preparation Time: 5 minutes

Cooking Time: 20 minutes

Servings: 5 servings

Ingredients:

- 1 cup chopped frozen spinach
- 1 egg
- ½ cup bread crumbs
- 4 Tbsp parmesan cheese
- 1 Tbsp butter, melted
- ¼ tsp ground black pepper
- ½ tsp salt
- ¼ tsp paprika

Instructions:

1. Defrost the frozen spinach and then press well in a strainer to remove all the excess water. The spinach should be very dry.
2. Place the spinach in a large bowl and mix all the other ingredients together in the bowl as well. Use your hands to really mix everything well.
3. Form into small balls, squeezing each with your hands. Place the balls on a lined sheet tray.
4. Bake the spinach balls for 15 minutes in a 350 degree oven. The bottoms should be nice and brown.
5. Enjoy warm.

Nutrition: Calories 99, fat 5g, fiber 1g, carbs 11g, protein 4g

Zucchini Pizza

Preparation Time: 5 minutes

Cooking Time: 15 minutes

Servings: 2 servings

Ingredients:

- 1 large zucchini
- ½ tsp Lowry's seasoning salt
- 1 tsp Italian seasoning
- ½ cup pizza sauce
- 1 cup shredded mozzarella

Instructions:

1. Slice the zucchini into 1/8 inch thick rounds, placing them on a sheet tray in a single layer as you slice.
2. Sprinkle the zucchini slices with the seasoning salt and Italian seasoning.
3. Spread the pizza sauce across the top of the zucchini.
4. Sprinkle the mozzarella across the zucchini as well.
5. Place the tray under a preheated broiler and bake for 5 minutes or until cheese begins to brown.
6. Remove from the broiler and serve warm.

Nutrition: Calories 88, fat 5g, fiber 3g, carbs 13g, protein 4g

Ants on a Log

Preparation Time: 5 minutes

Cooking Time: 0 minutes

Servings: 2 servings

Ingredients:

- 2 celery stalks, cut into 4" pieces
- ¼ cup peanut butter
- ¼ cup raisins

Instructions:

1. Place the celery strips on a plate.
2. Use a spoon to fill each piece celery with the peanut butter.
3. Place the raisins on top of the peanut butter, putting a nice row on raisins on each piece of celery.
4. Serve chilled

Nutrition: Calories 339, fat 16g, fiber 4g, carbs 46g, protein 9g

Broccoli Cheese Bread

Preparation Time: 15 minutes

Cooking Time: 30 minutes

Servings: 2 servings

Ingredients:

- 2 cups riced broccoli
- 1 egg
- 1 cup mozzarella cheese, shredded
- ¼ cup shredded cheddar cheese
- ½ tsp dried oregano
- ½ tsp salt
- 2 tsp fresh parsley

Instructions:

1. Microwave the riced broccoli on high for 1 minute to cook slightly. Press to remove any excess water and then place in a large bowl.
2. Add egg, half of the shredded cheeses, oregano and salt to the bowl with the broccoli and mix together well.
3. Place the batter on a lined sheet tray and spread until even and thin on the tray.
4. Place in a preheated 425 degree F oven and bake for 20 minutes.
5. Remove from the oven and sprinkle with the remaining cheeses. Return to the oven and bake for another 10 minutes or until the cheese begins to brown.
6. Remove from the oven, slice and serve warm.

Nutrition: Calories 463, fat 20g, fiber 0g, carbs 3g, protein 19g

Veggie Tart

Preparation Time: 5 minutes

Cooking Time: 15 minutes

Servings: 2 servings

Ingredients:

- 1 tbsp olive oil
- 1 large tomato, sliced
- ¼ tsp salt
- ¼ tsp ground black pepper
- 4 oz cream cheese
- ¼ cup chopped fresh basil
- 1 zucchini, sliced
- 1 pie crust

Instructions:

1. In a small bowl, mix together the cream cheese, basil, salt and pepper
2. Use a vegetable peeler to peel the zucchini into long strips.
3. Place the pie crust on a lined sheet tray.
4. Spread the cream cheese mix over the top of the pie crust evenly. Place the tomato slices on top of the cream cheese then top with the zucchini ribbons.
5. Fold the edge of the pie crust up, making a ½ inch border around the edge of the entire pie.
6. Brush the olive oil over the top of the pie, curst and veggies should be covered.
7. Bake for 30 minutes in a 425 degree F oven or until the edges of the pie crust begin to brown.
8. Serve warm.

Nutrition: Calories 693, fat 50g, fiber 2g, carbs 54g, protein 5g

Cheesy Kale Chips

Preparation Time: 5 minutes

Cooking Time: 45 minutes

Servings: 2 servings

Ingredients:

- 2 Tbsp olive oil or coconut oil
- 1 bunch kale, chopped
- ½ cup nutritional yeast
- 1/3 tsp salt

Instructions:

1. Place the kale in a large bowl and toss with the oil.
2. Add the nutritional yeast and salt and toss everything together well.
3. Transfer the mix to a lined sheet tray and place into a preheated 200 degree oven.
4. Bake for 20 minutes then toss the mixture on the tray. Bake for another 20 minutes.
5. Serve warm or room temperature

Nutrition: Calories 199, fat 15g, fiber 9g, carbs 20g, protein 18g

Coconut Carrots

Preparation Time: 5 minutes

Cooking Time: 20 minutes

Servings: 4 servings

Ingredients:

- 2 pounds carrots, chopped
- 1 can cream of coconut
- ¼ tsp salt
- ½ tsp vanilla extract

Instructions:

1. Add carrots and cream of coconut to a large sauce pan. Mix in salt and vanilla then heat over medium.
2. Simmer for 20 minutes or until the carrots are nice and tender. Serve warm.

Nutrition: Calories 516, fat 16g, fiber 6g, carbs 68g, protein 2g

Cauliflower Bites

Preparation Time: 15 minutes

Cooking Time: 30 minutes

Servings: 5 servings

Ingredients:

- 4 cups cauliflower florets
- 2 tbsp cornstarch
- 2 eggs, whisked
- 1 Tbsp whole milk
- 1 cup almond flour
- 1 cup grated parmesan cheese
- ½ tsp baking powder
- ½ tsp salt

Instructions:

1. Toss the cauliflower and cornstarch together in a large bowl.
2. In a separate bowl, combine the whisked egg, almond flour, baking powder, salt and cheese.
3. Toss the cauliflower in the egg mix, coating completely.
4. Transfer the coated cauliflower to a greased sheet tray and bake for 30 minutes in a 425 degree oven.
5. Remove from the oven when golden brown and serve warm

Nutrition: Calories 218, fat 15g, fiber 6g, carbs 12g, protein 10g

Beef Recipes

Spaghetti and Meatballs

Preparation Time: 10 minutes

Cooking Time: 30 minutes

Servings: 4 servings

Ingredients:

- 1 cup torn pieces of bread
- ¼ cup milk
- 1 ½ pounds ground beef
- 3 eggs
- 3 cloves garlic, minced
- 1 cup parmesan cheese, grated
- ½ cup fresh chopped parsley
- ½ tsp salt
- ½ tsp oregano
- ½ tsp ground black pepper
- 4 Tablespoons olive oil
- 1 pound spaghetti noodles, cooked
- 3 cups tomato sauce

Instructions:

1. Place bread and milk in a large bowl and let soak.
2. Add the beef, eggs, cheese, parsley, salt, oregano and black pepper and mix together well. Use your hands to really combine the meat.
3. Roll the meat mixture into golf ball sized meatballs, using your hands, then place them on a lined, rimmed baking sheet.
4. Add the olive oil to a large skillet and heat over medium high heat. Add the meatballs and cook for 5 minutes, turning occasionally just to brown the outside of the meatballs.
5. Add the tomato sauce to a large pot and bring to a simmer.
6. Add meatballs into the sauce and simmer, covered, for 15 minutes.
7. Divide the cooked spaghetti into 4 bowls and scoop the sauce and meatballs over the top. Serve while hot!

Nutrition: Calories 876, fat 45g, fiber 12g, carbs 85g, protein 45g

Beefy Grilled Cheese

Preparation Time: 15 minutes

Cooking Time: 10 minutes

Servings: 4 servings

Ingredients:

- 1 pound ground beef
- 1 tsp Lowry's Seasoning salt
- ¼ tsp ground black pepper
- 2 Tbsp oil
- 8 slices whole wheat bread
- 8 slices American cheese
- 4 Tbsp butter

Instructions:

1. In a large bowl, mix the beef, seasoning salt and black pepper together well. Divide into 4 and shape into patties.
2. Add the oil to a large pan and heat over medium. Add the beef patties and cook for 4 minutes, flip and cook for another 4 minutes. Remove the pan from the heat.
3. Place one burger on top of a piece of bread, then top with two pieces of cheese.
4. Place the other pieces of bread on top of the cheese, making a sandwich.
5. Add the butter to a large sauté pan and melt over low heat.
6. Add the sandwiches to the pan and cover. Cook for 3 minutes then flip the sandwiches, cook for three more minutes then serve warm.

Nutrition: Calories 487, fat 32g, fiber 1g, carbs 12g, protein 32g

Stuffed Burger

Preparation Time: 15 minutes

Cooking Time: 10 minutes

Servings: 4 servings

Ingredients:

- 1 pound ground beef
- ¼ tsp salt
- 2 Tbsp ketchup
- ½ tsp garlic powder
- ½ cup chopped bacon, cooked
- ¾ cup shredded cheddar cheese

Instruction:

1. In a large bowl, combine the beef, salt, ketchup, and garlic powder. Mix together well.
2. Shape the beef mixture into 4 large patties.
3. In a separate bowl, combine the cheese and bacon.
4. Hold one beef patty in your hand and make a large hole in the center of the patty, keeping the bottom in tact but shaping the patty into a bowl.
5. Scoop ¼ of the cheese mixture into the center of the flattened burger then wrap the beef over the cheese, shaping it back into a patty with the cheese and bacon hidden inside. Repeat with the remaining beef patties.
6. Cook the burgers on a preheated grill for 3 minutes on each side. Serve on a roll if desired while hot.

Nutrition: Calories 504, fat 22g, fiber 2g, carbs 24g, protein 43g

Sloppy Joes

Preparation Time: 10 minutes

Cooking Time: 16 minutes

Servings: 4 servings

Ingredients:

- 1 pound ground beef
- 1 ½ cups canned tomato soup
- 1/3 cup ketchup
- ½ onion, chopped
- ½ zucchini
- 1 tsp salt
- 1 tsp paprika
- 1 tbsp olive oil
- 4 burger buns

Instructions:

1. In a blender or a food processor, puree the onion and zucchini until smooth.
2. In a large skillet, heat the olive oil over medium heat.
3. Add the veggie puree to the pan and cook for 3 minutes.
4. Add the ground beef to the pan and season with the salt and paprika. Stir the mixture all together, breaking up the meat as it cooks and blending it in with the veggies. Cook for 5 minutes.
5. Add the tomato soup and ketchup to the pan and stir well. Cook for another 8 minutes, letting the mixture simmer.
6. Scoop the mixture onto the burger buns and serve while warm.

Nutrition: Calories 534, fat 27g, fiber 1g, carbs 35g, protein 39g

Taco Quesadillas

Preparation Time: 15 minutes

Cooking Time: 10 minutes

Servings: 4 servings

Ingredients:

- 1 pound ground beef
- 1 packet taco seasoning
- 2 cups shredded cheddar cheese
- 8 flour quesadillas

Instructions:

1. Place the ground beef in a skillet and cook over medium heat, breaking up the pieces of meat as it cooks. Cook until the meat is evenly browned, about 8 minutes.
2. Add the taco seasoning into the pan according to the instructions on the packet. Stir well then remove from the heat and let cool.
3. Add the shredded cheese to the taco meat and stir together.
4. Scoop the taco meat mixture onto the quesadillas and then fold the quesadillas in half.
5. Microwave each quesadilla for 30 seconds then serve while warm.

Nutrition: Calories 922, fat 54g, fiber 3g, carbs 45g, protein 56g

Cheeseburger Cups

Preparation Time: 15 minutes

Cooking Time: 15 minutes

Servings: 5 servings

Ingredients:

- 1 pound ground beef
- ½ cup ketchup
- 2 Tbsp brown sugar
- 2 tsp Worcestershire sauce
- 1 container (12 oz) refrigerated biscuit dough
- 1 cup cheddar cheese, shredded

Instructions:

1. In a medium sized skillet, brown the beef, stirring as you cook to break up the pieces. Drain any excess juice.
2. Add the ketchup to the pan along with the brown sugar and Worcestershire sauce. Stir well then remove from the heat.
3. Press each biscuit into a greased muffin tin, pushing the biscuit dough up the sides of the muffin cup.
4. Fill each muffin with the beef mixture then top with the shredded cheese.
5. Bake in a preheated 400 degree F oven for 15 minutes or until the cheese begins to bubble and turn golden brown.

Nutrition: Calories 467, fat 23g, fiber 1g, carbs 38g, protein 27g

Potato and Beef Cheese Cups

Preparation Time: 15 minutes

Cooking Time: 15 minutes

Servings: 4 servings

Ingredients:

- 1 pound ground beef
- ½ cup onion
- ½ cup ketchup
- 2 Tbsp brown sugar
- 2 tsp Worcestershire sauce
- ½ cup diced tomato
- 20 tater tots
- 1 cup cheddar cheese, shredded

Instructions:

1. In a medium sized skillet, brown the beef and onion, stirring as you cook to break up the pieces. Drain any excess juice.
2. Add the ketchup to the pan along with the brown sugar and Worcestershire sauce. Stir well then remove from the heat.
3. Stir in the diced tomato.
4. Grease a muffin tin and then place 4 tater tots in each muffin hole. Press the tater tots down, pressing them up the sides of the pan.
5. Fill the tater tot cups with the ground beef mixture then top with the cheese.
6. Bake in a 425 degree F oven for 15 minutes.
7. Remove the potato cups from the muffin tin and enjoy!

Nutrition: Calories 453, fat 24g, fiber 1g, carbs 31g, protein 32g

Chili Cheese "Hot Dogs"

Preparation Time: 15 minutes

Cooking Time: 25 minutes

Servings: 4 servings

Ingredients:

- 1 pound ground beef
- ½ cup diced onion
- 1 bell pepper, chopped
- 2 cloves garlic, minced
- 1 can (14 oz) fire roasted tomatoes, diced
- 1 Tbsp chili powder
- ½ tsp salt
- 4 hot dog rolls
- 1 cup shredded cheddar cheese

Instructions:

1. In a large skillet cook the ground beef, onion, bell pepper and garlic over medium heat. Stir occasionally, breaking up the pieces of beef. Cook until the meat has browned (about 8-10 minutes).
2. Add the fire roasted tomatoes and chili powder to the pan and stir. Bring to a simmer and then cook for another 10 minutes to thicken, stirring occasionally.
3. Scoop the beef mixture into the hot dog buns and sprinkle the cheese over the top.
4. Place the rolls on a sheet tray and under a preheated broiler for 2 minutes to melt the cheese.
5. Enjoy warm

Nutrition: Calories 518, fat 25g, fiber 5g, carbs 38g, protein 37g

BBQ Steak Kebobs

Preparation Time: 15 minutes

Cooking Time: 15 minutes

Servings: 4 servings

Ingredients:

- 1 pound steak tips (cut into 1" pieces)
- 20 cherry tomatoes
- 1 large onion, cut into 8 chunks
- ½ cup bbq sauce

Instructions:

1. Preheat your grill on high.
2. Skewer the steak tips, onion and tomatoes on 4 large skewers. Alternate the steak and veggies to make it extra pretty.
3. Brush each kebob with the BBQ sauce and then place directly on to the grill.
4. Cook for 4 minutes on one side then rotate the kebobs and cook for another 4 minutes.
5. Serve while hot with any extra BBQ sauce.

Nutrition: Calories 295, fat 7g, fiber 1g, carbs 33g, protein 24g

Mini Pizzas

Preparation Time: 15 minutes

Cooking Time: 15 minutes

Servings: 4 servings

Ingredients:

- 2 english muffins, slit in half
- ½ cup pizza sauce
- ½ pound ground beef
- 1 Tbsp Worcestershire sauce
- ¼ tsp salt
- ½ cup mozzarella cheese

Instructions:

1. Cook the beef in a large skillet over medium heat until it is browned (about 10 minutes). Break the beef up with a spatula as it cooks.
2. Stir in the salt and Worcestershire sauce.
3. Place the English Muffins on a plate with the hole side up.
4. Spread the pasta sauce over each English muffin.
5. Sprinkle each muffin with the cooked beef.
6. Sprinkle the cheese on each mini pizza, covering the beef.
7. Place the pizzas on a sheet tray and place under a preheated broiler for 3 minutes or until the cheese begins to bubble and brown.
8. Serve while warm!

Nutrition: Calories 380, fat 20g, fiber 2g, carbs 19g, protein 32g

Salad Recipes

Kale and Carrot Salad

Preparation Time: 10 minutes

Cooking Time: 15 minutes

Servings: 4 servings

Ingredients:

- 4 cups kale, chopped very small
- 1 Tbsp olive oil
- 2 carrots, shredded
- 1 small zucchini, shredded
- ½ tsp salt
- ½ cup water
- ½ cup raisins
- 1 cup feta cheese, crumbled

Instructions:

1. In a large skillet, add the olive oil and heat over medium.
2. Add the kale, zucchini and carrot to the pan and stir.
3. Add in the salt, pepper and water. Cover the pan and cook for 10 minutes to wilt the kale.
4. Remove from the heat and let cool.
5. Add he cheese and raisins then toss together.
6. Serve chilled.

Nutrition: Calories 245, fat 12g, fiber 7g, carbs 32g, protein 12g

Squash and Quinoa Salad

Preparation Time: 5 minutes

Cooking Time: 0 minutes

Servings: 4 servings

Ingredients:

- 1/3 cup mayonnaise
- 2 Tbsp apple cider vinegar
- 1 tsp brown sugar
- 4 cups broccoli florets
- ½ cup dried cranberries
- ½ cup bell pepper, diced

Instructions:

1. In a small bowl, mix together the mayo, vinegar and sugar.
2. In a large bowl, toss together the broccoli, pepper and cranberries.
3. Add the dressing to the broccoli mix and toss well to coat.
4. Chill in the fridge for one hour then serve.

Nutrition: Calories 268, fat 14g, fiber 5g, carbs 34g, protein 2g

Kale and Carrot Salad

Preparation Time: 5 minutes

Cooking Time: 10 minutes

Servings: 4 servings

Ingredients:

- ½ cup quinoa, cooked
- 2 Tbsp olive Oil
- 1 pound butternut squash, peeled and chopped into 1 inch pieces
- ¼ tsp salt
- ¼ cup apple cider vinegar
- 3 Tbsp tahini paste
- 1 Tbsp honey
- 4 cups arugula

Instructions:

1. Add olive oil to a large skillet and add the squash. Saute for 10 minutes or until the squash is browned and tender.
2. Add salt and cook for one more minute.
3. In a small bowl, mix together the cider vinegar, tahini, honey and olive oil in a bowl and whisk well.
4. Place arugula in a bowl and toss with the dressing. Add the squash and toss more.
5. Divide between plates and serve

Nutrition: Calories 252, fat 17g, fiber 16g, carbs 68g, protein 4g

Watermelon Cucumber Salad

Preparation Time: 5 minutes

Cooking Time: 0 minutes

Servings: 5 servings

Ingredients:

- 4 cups watermelon chunks
- 1 large cucumber, peeled and sliced
- 1 Tbsp olive oil
- 1 Tbsp balsamic vinegar
- ¼ tsp salt
- One inch of black pepper
- 1 Tbsp chopped mint
- 2 Tbsp pepita seeds

Instructions:

1. In a large bowl, combine the watermelon and cucumber.
2. Add the remaining ingredients and toss together well.
3. Serve chilled

Nutrition: Calories 103, fat 5g, fiber 1g, carbs 15g, protein 2g

Crunchy Apple Salad

Preparation Time: 5 minutes

Cooking Time: 0 minutes

Servings: 2 servings

Ingredients:

- 1/3 cup plain yogurt
- 2 Tbsp mayonnaise
- 2 tbsp lime juice
- 1 tsp honey
- ¼ tsp salt
- 1 pinch ground black pepper
- 2 large apples, sliced
- 1 cup chopped celery
- 1 cup chopped cucumber

Instructions:

1. In a small bowl, whisk together the yogurt, mayo, lime juice, honey. Salt and pepper.
2. In a large bowl, combine the apples, celery and cucumber.
3. Pour the dressing over the salad and toss.
4. Serve chilled

Nutrition: Calories 103, fat 4g, fiber 1g, carbs 12g, protein 3g

Chicken Mango Salad

Preparation Time: 15 minutes

Cooking Time: 0 minutes

Servings: 4 servings

Ingredients:

- 8 cups romaine lettuce
- 2 mangos, peeled and sliced
- ¼ cup red onion, sliced
- 1 pound grilled chicken breast, sliced
- 4 Tbsp olive oil
- 2 tbsp lime juice
- ¼ cup orange juice
- 1 tsp sugar
- ¼ tsp salt
- ¼ cup cilantro, chopped

Instructions:

1. In a large bowl, toss the lettuce, mango, onion and chicken together.
2. In a separate small bowl, add the olive oil, lime juice, orange juice, sugar and salt. Whisk together then pour over the salad.
3. Toss everything together well and serve.

Nutrition: Calories 352, fat 22g, fiber 3g, carbs 22g, protein 16g

Finger Food Salad

Preparation Time: 10 minutes

Cooking Time: 5 minutes

Servings: 5 servings

Ingredients

- 2 cups frozen edamame, shells removed
- 1 can black beans, drained and rinsed
- 2 oranges, peeled, segmented and chopped
- 1 cup pomegranate seeds
- 1 Tbsp rice vinegar
- 2 Tbsp orange juice
- 1 Tbsp olive oil
- 1 tsp honey
- 1 pinch salt
- 1 pinch black pepper

Instructions:

1. Boil edamame in water for 5 minutes. Drain and rinse with cold water then place in a large bowl.
2. Add the black beans, orange segments and pomegranate seeds to the bowl as well and toss together.
3. In a small bowl, whisk together the remaining ingredients to make a dressing and then pour over the salad.
4. Toss well and serve.

Nutrition: Calories 297, fat 7g, fiber 10g, carbs 42g, protein 14g

Cucumber Salad

Preparation Time: 10 minutes

Cooking Time: 5 minutes

Servings: 5 servings

Ingredients

- 1 Tbsp shallots, minced
- 1 Tbsp white wine vinegar
- 1 Tbsp olive oil
- ½ tsp sugar
- ¼ tsp salt
- 5 cups chopped cucumber
- 1 Tbsp chopped mint

Instructions:

1. In a large bowl, combine the shallots, vinegar, olive oil, sugar. Salt and pepper. Whisk together.
2. Add the cucumbers to the bowl and toss well.
3. Sprinkle with the mint and serve chilled.

Nutrition: Calories 52, fat 4g, fiber 2g, carbs 4g, protein 1g

Wheat Berry Salad

Preparation Time: 25 minutes

Cooking Time: 65 minutes

Servings: 5 servings

Ingredients

- 2 cups wheat berries
- 4 cups water
- 1/3 cup olive oil
- 3 Tbsp orange juice
- 1 tsp fresh grated orange zest
- 2 Tbsp honey
- 1 tsp salt
- ¼ tsp ground black pepper
- ½ cup chopped almonds
- 1 cup chopped orange segments
- 1 cup chopped celery
- 1 cup chopped dried apricots
- ¼ cup chopped fresh parsley
- ¼ cup chopped fresh mint

Instructions:

1. Add wheat berries to a pot along with the water and bring to a boil. Cover and simmer over low heat for one hour or until the berries are tender and chewy. Pour off any extra water then cool the cooked wheat berries
2. In a large bowl, whisk together the oil, balsamic, orange zest, honey, salt and pepper.
3. Add the wheat berries to the bowl and toss in the dressing.
4. Add the remaining ingredients and toss again. Serve chilled or slightly warm

Nutrition: Calories 367, fat 17g, fiber 6g, carbs 47g, protein 7g

Arugula Watermelon Salad

Preparation Time: 15 minutes

Cooking Time: 0 minutes

Servings: 4 servings

Ingredients

- ½ cup orange juice
- ¼ cup shallots, minced
- 1 Tbsp honey
- 6 Tbsp olive oil
- 1 tsp salt
- 6 cups baby arugula
- 2 cups chopped watermelon
- 1 cup feta cheese
- ½ cup chopped fresh mint

Instructions:

1. In a large bowl, whisk together the orange juice, shallots, honey, olive oil and salt.
2. Add the remaining ingredients to the bowl with the dressing and toss well.
3. Serve chilled

Nutrition: Calories 301, fat 31g, fiber 1g, carbs 26g, protein 8g

Snack Recipes

Chocolate Chip Banana Sandwich

Preparation Time: 10 minutes

Cooking Time: 0 minutes

Servings: 2 servings

Ingredients:

- ¼ cup peanut butter
- 2 Tbsp honey
- ¼ tsp cinnamon
- 2 Tbsp mini chocolate chips
- 4 pieces whole wheat bread
- 1 banana, sliced

Instructions;

1. In a small bowl, mix together the peanut butter, honey and cinnamon.
2. Spread the peanut butter mix over the bread
3. Add the banana sliced on top of each piece of bread.
4. Enjoy!

Nutrition: Calories 502, fat 20g, fiber 7g, carbs 64g, protein 13g

Chocolate Granola Pretzel Sticks

Preparation Time: 15 minutes

Cooking Time: 0 minutes

Servings: 5 servings

Ingredients:

- 1 ½ cups chocolate chips
- 10 pretzel rods
- 1 cup granola

Instructions:

1. Place the chocolate chips in a tall microwave safe glass. Microwave for 20 seconds at a time, stirring after each microwave to prevent the chocolate from burning. Microwave until the chips have melted and the chocolate is smooth.
2. Place the granola on a plate.
3. Dip each pretzel rod in the chocolate and then roll in the granola.
4. Set on a tray to let the chocolate harden and then enjoy!

Nutrition: Calories 242, fat 10g, fiber 4g, carbs 35g, protein 6g

Peanut Butter Balls

Preparation Time: 10 minutes

Cooking Time: 0 minutes

Servings: 5 servings

Ingredients:

- ¼ cup peanut butter
- 2 Tbsp honey
- ¼ tsp vanilla extract
- ¼ cup dry milk powder
- ¼ cup rolled oats
- ¼ cup mini chocolate chips

Instructions:

1. In a bowl, mix together the peanut butter, vanilla and honey.
2. Add the remaining ingredients and stir well.
3. Scoop the dough into one inch balls and roll together with your hands.
4. Place the balls on a tray and refrigerate until ready to eat.

Nutrition: Calories 70, fat 3g, fiber 1g, carbs 9g, protein 3g

Crunchy Snack Mix

Preparation Time: 10 minutes

Cooking Time: 0 minutes

Servings: 5 servings

Ingredients:

- 1 cup animal crackers
- 1 cup mini pretzels
- 1 cup salted peanuts
- 1 cup mini chocolate chips
- 1 cup chocolate covered raisins

Instructions:

1. Add all the ingredients to a large bowl and toss together. Scoop into bowls and enjoy!

Nutrition: Calories 266, fat 14g, fiber 3g, carbs 33g, protein 6g

Peanut Butter Pinwheels

Preparation Time: 5 minutes

Cooking Time: 0 minutes

Servings: 2 servings

Ingredients:

- 2 Tbsp peanut butter, creamy or chunky
- 1 flour tortilla
- 2 tsp honey
- ½ cup granola with raisins

Instructions:

1. Place the tortilla on a flat work surface.
2. Spread the peanut butter on the tortilla.
3. Drizzle the tortilla with the honey and then top with the granola.
4. Roll the tortilla up and then cut into slices

Nutrition: Calories 60, fat 3g, fiber 1g, carbs 7g, protein 2g

PBJ Fruit Sticks

Preparation Time: 10 minutes

Cooking Time: 0 minutes

Servings: 4 servings

Ingredients:

- 2 PBJ Sandwiches
- 1 cup grapes
- 1 cup strawberry halves

Instructions:

1. Cut each sandwich into 4 pieces
2. Place one piece of PBJ on a wooden skewer followed by a grape, one strawberry half and then repeat.
3. Make 4 skewers, each with 2 pieces of PBJ.
4. Enjoy immediately!

Nutrition: Calories 205, fat 6g, fiber 4g, carbs 31g, protein 6g

Ranch Snack Mix

Preparation Time: 15 minutes

Cooking Time: 0 minutes

Servings: 5 servings

Ingredients:

- 2 cups mini pretzels
- 2 cups bugels
- 1 cup salted cashews
- 1 cup goldfish crackers
- 1 package ranch salad dressing mix
- ½ cup olive oil

Instructions:

1. Add the pretzels, bugels, cashews and goldfish crackers to a large bowl and toss together.
2. Sprinkle with the ranch mix then drizzle with the oil and toss.
3. Serve at room temperature.

Nutrition: Calories 185, fat 11g, fiber 1g, carbs 19g, protein 4g

Apple Peanut Butter Sandwiches

Preparation Time: 10 minutes

Cooking Time: 0 minutes

Servings: 5 servings

Ingredients:

- 2 apples, cored and sliced
- 1/3 cup peanut butter, smooth or chunky
- ½ cup mini M&M's

Instructions:

1. Spread the peanut butter across the top of half the apple slices.
2. Sprinkle the apple slices with the mini M&M's.
3. Top each sandwich with another apple slice and enjoy!

Nutrition: Calories 145, fat 8g, fiber 2g, carbs 19g, protein 2g

Peach Berry Bowl

Preparation Time: 10 minutes

Cooking Time: 0 minutes

Servings: 4 servings

Ingredients:

- 2 peaches, pitted and sliced
- ¼ cup honey
- 1 tsp lemon juice
- 3 oz cream cheese
- 1 cup raspberries
- 1 cup blueberries

Instructions:

1. In a small bowl, mix together the peaches, honey and lemon juice. Place in fridge for one hour.
2. Drain the juice from the peaches into a small bowl and add the cream cheese to the juice. Mix together well until incorporated fully and smooth.
3. Add the berries to the peaches and toss together.
4. Divide the peaches and berries into four bowls and top with the cream cheese mix. Serve cold.

Nutrition: Calories 109, fat 3g, fiber 4g, carbs 21g, protein 2g

Blueberry Dip

Preparation Time: 10 minutes

Cooking Time: 0 minutes

Servings: 2 servings

Ingredients:

- ½ cup cream cheese
- ¼ cup powdered sugar
- ½ tsp cinnamon
- 1 tsp lemon juice
- ½ cup fresh blueberries
- 1 cup graham crackers
- 1 cup sliced apples

Instructions:

1. Beat the cream cheese, powdered sugar, cinnamon and lemon juice together until fluffy and smooth.
2. Gently mix in the blueberries, folding easily so they do not break.
3. Serve the dip with the graham crackers and fruit.

Nutrition: Calories 84, fat 3g, fiber 2g, carbs 9g, protein 1g

Dessert Recipes

Icebox Ice Cream Sandwiches

Preparation Time: 20 minutes

Cooking Time: 0 minutes

Servings: 5 servings

Ingredients:

- 1 package Instant vanilla pudding
- 2 cups whole milk, cold
- 2 cups Cool Whip
- 1 cup mini chocolate chips
- 10 graham crackers

Instructions:

1. Make the pudding using the cold milk according to the package directions. Refrigerate until the pudding has set
2. Add the chocolate chips and cool whip to the pudding and fold together well.
3. Place the graham crackers on a sheet tray and top half of them with the pudding mix.
4. Sandwich another graham cracker on top of the pudding then place all the sandwiches in the freezer until firm, about 3 hours.
5. Enjoy cold!

Nutrition: Calories 144, fat 5g, fiber 1g, carbs 3g, protein 2g

Mini Monkey Treats

Preparation Time: 20 minutes

Cooking Time: 0 minutes

Servings: 5 servings

Ingredients:

- 2 bananas
- 1 cup chocolate chips
- 1 tsp coconut oil
- ¼ cup shredded coconut
- ¼ cup chopped peanuts

Instructions:

1. Cut the bananas into 5 pieces and place a toothpick into each slice. Place the banana slices on a lined sheet tray and place into the freezer for at least an hour.
2. In a microwave safe bowl, melt the chocolate chips and coconut oil together, microwaving for 20 seconds at a time and stirring every time.
3. Place the coconut and peanuts into a bowl and mix together
4. Dip the frozen bananas into the melted chocolate and then into the coconut and peanut mix. Place on a sheet tray to harden.
5. Enjoy cold!

Nutrition: Calories 140, fat 4g, fiber 2g, carbs 20g, protein 2g

Raspberry Ice Cream

Preparation Time: 15 minutes

Cooking Time: 0 minutes

Servings: 2 servings

Ingredients:

- 1 cup cream
- ½ cup raspberries
- ¼ cup sugar
- 2 Tbsp evaporated milk
- ½ tsp vanilla

Instructions:

1. In a small Ziploc bag, add all of the ingredients and seal closed.
2. In a large, gallon sized Ziploc bag, add 4 cups of ice and ¾ cup salt.
3. Place the small bag into the large bag with the ice. Seal the large bag closed.
4. Shake and press the small bag until it has thickened. It should take about 5 minutes of shaking to thicken.
5. Open the small bag and scoop the ice cream into dishes and enjoy

Nutrition: Calories 150, fat 5g, fiber 1g, carbs 17g, protein 3g

S'Mores Casserole

Preparation Time: 10 minutes

Cooking Time: 20 minutes

Servings: 5 servings

Ingredients:

- 2 cups marshmallows
- 6 chocolate bars, broken into pieces
- 20 graham crackers

Instructions:

1. Grease a casserole dish them place half the marshmallows in the pan.
2. Top with the half the chocolate pieces and half the graham cracker pieces.
3. Repeat layering.
4. Place in a preheated 400 degree oven and bake for 10 minutes or until the marshmallows turn golden brown.
5. Allow to cool for a few minutes then enjoy.

Nutrition: Calories 247, fat 6g, fiber 1g, carbs 45g, protein 3g

Puppy Chow

Preparation Time: 15 minutes

Cooking Time: 0 minutes

Servings: 5 servings

Ingredients:

- 1 cup mini chocolate chips
- ½ cup peanut butter
- 4 Tbsp butter, melted
- 1 tsp vanilla
- ¼ tsp salt
- 8 cups chex cereal
- 2 cups powdered sugar

Instructions:

1. Add the chocolate chips, peanut butter and melted butter to a microwave safe bowl and microwave for one minute. Stir to blend the mix together well and microwave more until smooth. Add the vanilla and mix again.
2. Add the chex into a large bowl and pour the chocolate mix over the top. Toss until all the cereal is coated in the chocolate.
3. Pour the powdered sugar into the bowl and toss again.
4. Let the puppy chow cool and then enjoy!

Nutrition: Calories 578, fat 23g, fiber 3g, carbs 84g, protein 9g

Waffle S'Mores

Preparation Time: 5 minutes

Cooking Time: 10 minutes

Servings: 5 servings

Ingredients:

- 10 mini waffles
- 10 chocolate squares
- 10 marshmallows
- 2 Tbsp cinnamon sugar

Instructions:

1. Place 5 of the mini waffle on a lined sheet tray.
2. Place one piece of chocolate and one marshmallow on top of each waffle.
3. Top the marshmallow with the rest of the mini waffles, making a sandwich.
4. Sprinkle with the cinnamon sugar then place into a preheated 400 degree oven for 4 minutes.
5. Press down gently on the top mini waffle to flatten and enjoy while warm.

Nutrition: Calories 607, fat 26g, fiber 3g, carbs 113g, protein 5g

Chocolate Popcorn

Preparation Time: 15 minutes

Cooking Time: 0 minutes

Servings: 4 servings

Ingredients:

- 1 bag microwave popcorn
- 2 cups white chocolate chips
- 1 tsp coconut oil
- 1 cup rainbow sprinkles

Instructions:

1. Pop the popcorn according to the directions. Then place the cooked popcorn in a large bowl.
2. In a microwave safe bowl, cook the white chocolate chips and coconut oil, microwaving for 20 seconds at a time, stirring every time, until the chocolate is melted and smooth.
3. Pour the melted chocolate over the popcorn and toss quickly.
4. Add the sprinkles and toss again.
5. Chill before serving

Nutrition: Calories 847, fat 47g, fiber 1g, carbs 113g, protein 1g

Banana Spilt Pops

Preparation Time: 15 minutes

Cooking Time: 0 minutes

Servings: 4 servings

Ingredients:

- 2 bananas
- ½ cup melted chocolate chips
- 1 Tsp coconut oil
- ¼ cup rainbow sprinkles
- Whipped cream
- 4 cherries

Instructions:

1. Peel and slice each banana. Place a popsicle stick into each banana and place the bananas in the freezer.
2. Whisk the coconut oil into the melted chocolate.
3. Place the sprinkles in a small bowl.
4. Dip the bananas into the chocolate and then into the sprinkles. Place on a tray to harden.
5. When ready to eat, squirt some whipped cream on top of the bananas and to with a cherry. Enjoy cold!

Nutrition: Calories 293, fat 12g, fiber 4g, carbs 45g, protein 3g

Ice Cream Brownie Cups

Preparation Time: 15 minutes

Cooking Time: 25 minutes

Servings: 5 servings

Ingredients:

- ½ box brownie mix
- 2 cups ice cream
- Rainbow sprinkles

Ingredients:

1. Prepare the brownie mix according to the package directions.
2. Spray a muffin tin with non stick spray then scoop the brownie batter into the muffin cups.
3. Bake for 25 minutes according to the brownie package. Remove from the oven and use the bottom of a small glass to press down the center of the brownies, making them into a cup. Then let cool.
4. Place one brownie on each plate and scoop the ice cream into the cup. Top with sprinkles and serve.

Nutrition: Calories 177, fat 9g, fiber 1g, carbs 22g, protein 3g

Peanut Butter Rice Krispie Treats

Preparation Time: 20 minutes

Cooking Time: 10 minutes

Servings: 5 servings

Ingredients:

- 3 Tbsp butter
- 2 cups mini marshmallows
- 4 Tbsp peanut butter
- 3 cups rice krispies
- ¼ cup mini chocolate chips

Ingredients:

1. Grease a 8x8 inch pan.
2. In a large saucepan, melt the butter over low heat.
3. Add the marshmallows to the pan and stir constantly until they are melted. Add the peanut butter and stir into the mixture.
4. Remove from the heat and add the rice krispies and chocolate chips and stir quickly and thoroughly.
5. Pour the mix into the prepared pan and press down to make the treats even.
6. Allow to cool then remove from the pan, slice and serve.

Nutrition: Calories 270, fat 14g, fiber 1g, carbs 33g, protein 5g

CPSIA information can be obtained
at www.ICGtesting.com
Printed in the USA
LVHW101927080321
680894LV00012B/113